CW01335692

Reverse Type 2 Diabetes Naturally

Change the Quality of Your Life With Nutrition and Add Healthy Years

by

Marie Minani

ISBN: 978-1-914933-50-9

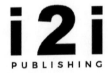

i2i Publishing. Manchester.
www.i2ipublishing.co.uk

Disclaimer

The aim of this book is to provide information only and should not be used as a substitute for the medical advice of your doctor or any other healthcare professional. The publisher and Author are not responsible or liable for any diagnosis made by a reader based on the contents of this book. Always consult your doctor if you are concerned about your health.

Author

Marie studied BSc. (Hons) Human Biology and Infectious diseases at the University of Salford 2012. Her research included type 2 diabetes with a special interest in nutrition. Passionate about what we eat, she later trained in Pg. Cert Human Nutrition at Manchester Metropolitan University 2021.

Acknowledgements

My profound gratitude and love as always go to Anthony Ronald Lawton who is always such a source of inspiration, support and understanding when I'm under pressure.

My warmest thanks to Lionel Ross for your valued advice and for reading the manuscript. I highly appreciate all the team at i2i Publishing who made the experience of writing this book possible.

I am forever grateful to Prof. Geoff Hide from the School of Environmental Life Sciences at the University of Salford who helped me build interest in the study.

I must acknowledge Haleh Moravej, Senior Lecturer in Nutritional Sciences at Manchester Metropolitan University, for delivering quality lectures and my personal life experiences that have urged me to accomplish writing this book.

Contents

Chapter 1: Introduction

There has been an increasing number of people developing type 2 diabetes in the United Kingdom (UK) and worldwide. Diabetes is a chronic disease that raises blood sugar levels but it does not have to be permanent. Treatments are evidence based on a low carbohydrate diet, stress reduction strategies, supplements, and recipes for reversing type 2 diabetes. I am passionate about reversing type 2 diabetes as it is personal to me since my sister had type 2 diabetes at an early age of forty years. Unfortunately, she didn't know how to change her lifestyle and lost her life after fourteen years of pain. In 2019, after that traumatic situation, I was eating junk food and not having much sleep. After a blood test at my surgery, I was told that I had pre-diabetes and had fatty liver; my heart was pounding. So, I started researching and put what I studied into action. After three months of changing my lifestyle, I managed to reverse pre-diabetes and reversed fatty liver after one year. Since 2019, I have eaten low carbohydrate foods mainly, reduced stress by doing simple exercises like walking, Tai Chi and stayed healthy. I sleep seven to eight hours every night and type 2 diabetes has been in remission up to today.

I am writing this book to help others so that they do not too feel helpless. I realized that food is a powerful medicine; when you eat the right food, you can optimize your health. We have all heard the phrase "let food be thy medicine" by Hippocrates, the father of all medicine. So, it is important to eat healthy foods, mainly vegetables, less tropical fruits, fish and organic meat. There are supplements you can take if that is what you prefer made from liver and other animal organs. If you are a vegan or vegetarian, there are alternative supplements you can take made from herbs, such as milk thistle and dandelion burdock root with a full glass of water. A diet high in nutrients has healing properties. Most people get much more energy; adrenal glands are strengthened, and it helps people to recover.

Foods high in sugar and refined carbohydrates will raise blood sugar levels and you may get depressed or irritable. It is undeniable that we live in stressful times; many of us have to cope with financial worries, emotional stress, the breakup of close relationships and bereavement.

This book will educate you, and you will benefit from my many years of research and enjoy healthier and happier lives.

Symptoms

According to the Mayo Clinic, people with type 2 diabetes might have no symptoms at all or few symptoms for years before being diagnosed. Some of the health issues people with type 2 diabetes develop include: frequent urination, infections, excessive thirst, difficulty in concentrating, excessive sweating, extreme difficulty in getting out of bed, falling asleep in the middle of the day, inability to get going without caffeine, hunger, slow wound healing, blurred vision, kidney disease, heart diseases, stroke, dental diseases, nerve damage, numbness in fingers, toes, pain in the feet, vision loss and coma.

Chapter 2: Diagnosis

Laboratory tests are essential for diagnosing diabetes, such as Fasting plasma glucose (FPG). Harvard Medical School suggests the test is done after fasting overnight; blood is taken from the patient's vein, in order to check blood sugar levels. Normal blood glucose should be from 70 to 100 milligrams per deciliter (mg/dl). When fasting blood glucose is 126 mg per deciliter and above that number confirms that a person has developed diabetes.

The American Diabetes Association advised that an Oral glucose tolerance test (OGTT) should be used to diagnose people with type 2 diabetes. The patient is asked to drink 75 grams of glucose; then blood sugar levels are tested every two hours and a reading of 200mg per dl or above indicates diabetes. A test known as HbA1C which determines approximate of metabolic control over a previous period of two to three months is also used to diagnose type 2 diabetes. Routine medical tests will be done for obese people or individuals with high blood pressure mainly aged 45 years and older with Body Mass Index (BMI) higher than 25kg/m2.

A Report by the National Institute of Health (NIH) states that type 2 diabetes is not necessarily a disease of obese individuals. The American study showed only 28% of obese people have type 2 diabetes. Diabetes is common in some ethnicities; an example is black people due to lifestyle choices. Where we were born impacts our mindset, and generations may shape our history. We are all human beings, but some people are more susceptible to diabetes despite having normal body mass index (BMI) due to genetic effect. Another example is people from South Asia and the Far East, they may seem to appear skinny but could be clinically obese. The term for that is known as (TOFI) which means thin on the outside fat inside. Thin individuals with high levels of visceral fat need to be concerned about their health. Many may not change their lifestyles as they might not know about hidden dangers beneath their skin.

The World Health Organization (WHO) estimates that by the year 2030, nearly three-quarters of men and two-thirds of women will be overweight. That will have a negative impact on people's health and the nation's economy. It is necessary to have an early diagnosis so that the condition can be reversed sooner than later. It can be achieved by less expensive methods such as monitoring blood sugar levels, physical activity, eating low carbohydrate foods and losing excess weight.

Chapter 3: Management & Treatment

Clinical intervention may be needed when a patient's blood sugar levels are unstable. Many doctors prescribe medication for type 2 diabetes such as Metformin as the first choice of treatment. It lowers blood sugar levels, yet the liver produces excess sugar in the body which reduces the production of a hormone called insulin. There are other groups of medication that help in filtering the kidneys too. Furthermore, treatments depend on the condition of an individual patient and the advice of the health care professionals.

The body pumps out glucose all the time, it does not come from food alone and fat in the pancreas can stop the pancreas from producing enough insulin. Then an excess amount of fat in the liver indicates that a person has insulin resistance. Researchers from Newcastle University in England observed that in clinical settings, eating low carbohydrate diets and fewer calories provided more benefits in decreasing total cholesterol, reduction in medication dependence, weight loss and blood sugar levels.

An average measure of a blood test after a period of three months is recommended to check the amount of blood sugar (glucose) that is attached on the hemoglobin. The hemoglobin is the part of your red blood cells that carries oxygen from the lungs to the rest of the body. The blood test is important to indicate how well your diabetes is being controlled. When the blood sugar level is 6.5% or 48mmol/mol it determines a person has diabetes or is at risk of developing type 2 diabetes. Individuals should aim at a blood test result showing of 6% level or 42mmol/mol free from medication before you can confirm that someone is free from type 2 diabetes.

In 2011, a report found that up to 24,000 people with diabetes in England lose their lives earlier from causes that could have been avoided through better management of their condition. Fortunately, while you can be genetically predisposed to type 2 diabetes, it is mostly caused by lifestyle factors. In fact, according to diabetes researcher Richard Beliveau, adopting a healthy lifestyle can prevent up to 90 per cent of type 2 cases. A landmark study sponsored by the National Institute of Health stated that to lose 5 to 7 per cent of your body weight is all the fat you need to shave in order to enjoy a nearly 60 per cent reduction in risk of type 2 diabetes; you make also exercise 150 minutes each week.

Exercise is the most significant step you can take to fight diabetes, one that is of even greater effect than the popular anti-diabetic drug metformin. Walking two and a half hours a week increased physical activity was one of the ways participants in the study reduced their risk of diabetes. It requires two 30 minutes of walking or other exercise of moderate intensity, five days per week. Stay committed and block off half an hour on your daily schedule as you would do any other important appointment. The other way participants succeeded was to eat low calorie and low fat; a diet rich in whole grains, fruits and vegetables can lower diabetes by 34 per cent.

Just one fizzy drink a day, whether regular or diet, has been linked 44 per cent greater chance of developing metabolic diseases, a collection of risk factors for diabetes and cardiovascular disease. Be happy; depression is another factor that causes diabetes. The same study showed that altered body chemistry raised insulin resistance by 23 per cent among women.

The fastest way to lower insulin levels is to substitute refined carbohydrate foods with moderate fats and proteins. The best choice of foods are fatty fish such as wild salmon, vegetables, green leafy foods, cauliflower, broccoli, kale, sweet potatoes occasionally, papaya, pumpkin, parsley, watercress, carrots, beet greens, dandelion greens, olive oil, avocadoes, raw nuts and seeds.

Foods and drinks that stabilize Blood Sugar

There are factors to bear in mind regarding keeping blood sugar levels stable; how regular you eat, and the nature of food you eat. The Mediterranean diet is considered to be the best by nutritionists; foods consumed include beans, salads, brown rice, seeds, eggs, fresh fruits, vegetables, poultry, skinless turkey, healthy fats such as cold-pressed olive oil, Avocado oil, unsweetened yoghurt, raw nuts (avoid salted or roasted nuts), fish like salmon, sardines, herring, mackerel, tuna are good in good fats called omega 3, essential for reducing cholesterol. Eat freshwater white fish baked or boiled (avoid fried fish), portions of red meat, lamb occasionally, mineral water, and unsweetened and herbal teas. Those foods are high in fibre with slow absorption of carbohydrates, and they keep you full for longer, which improves health and well-being.

This can be done by anyone who decides to change their lifestyle including people from low socioeconomic backgrounds. The international guidelines on dietary management of type 2 diabetes support carbohydrate restriction as a therapeutic strategy.

Therefore, be kind to yourself: do not consume over-processed foods, eat your greens to balance your blood sugar, get a good night's sleep, reduce stress, limit alcohol intake, and do some relaxing exercises. The good news is that making some changes to what we eat, how we move and the thoughts we think can have a positive impact on our physical and mental health. What to expect when you change your lifestyles to reverse type 2 diabetes include: increased energy, improved blood pressure, improved cholesterol levels, your heart becomes stronger, increased lifespan, improved immune system, reduced stress and learn how to make healthy delicious recipes.

More efficient food fuel for the body, Some examples:

Healthy recipes, green smoothies:
Fill one cup of frozen kale in a blender
Add one cup of your favourite berries either blue, black, or strawberries
300 ml water
One kiwi fruit / or a squeeze of lemon to taste
Combine all the ingredients in a blender and whip until smooth.
Take it at lunchtime or dinner.
Choice: 2
1 cup of low-fat yogurt mixed with a hand full of berries
Option: 3
2 servings
Baked skinless salmon fillets or Haddock, 1cm in thickness
A tablespoon of olive oil or melted butter
A clove of garlic minced, 1/8 ground black pepper, a tablespoon lemon juice, a pinch of salt
A tablespoon of chopped parsley
Mix all the above ingredients in a bowl and bake for 15 minutes until the fish is cooked through, on gas mark 6 or electricity 200C. Serve with vegetables of your choice such as cabbage, peas, carrots, broccoli or green beans.
Salad options
2 cups grilled skinless chicken breast chunks or alternatively boiled eggs
¼ cup fresh finely chopped basil, ½ cup fresh finely chopped celery and 3 cups mixed salad greens; aim at

rainbow yellow, red, and purple colours such as tomatoes, red cabbage, peppers, rockets and any seasonal organic vegetables

Combine all ingredients, substitute salt with vinegar and pepper or a tablespoon of lemon juice.

Mix well and enjoy your meal.

Chapter 4: Foods and Drinks that spike Blood Sugar

The foods that should be cut down and foods that you may be cut out completely include puddings, cookies, table sugar, white bread, sweets, fizzy drinks, sodas, pastries, squashes, alcohol, mashed potatoes and all junk foods. An example would be tinned foods such as tomato soup which contains artificial colours or preservatives.

Managing to control blood sugar levels is very important in order to avoid damage to the vital organs of your body. Some patients can get a condition called hypoglycemia, a sign of low blood sugar which include dizziness, trembling, sweating, fast heartbeat, kidney disease, nerve damage, limb amputation, mental health issues, oral health problems, and vision and hearing loss.

Foods to avoid

Crisps, white bread, potato chips, pasta, biscuits, chocolate bars, soda, coca colas, ginger beer, alcohol, energy drinks and cakes. Those foods cause the metabolism to become weak and fat burning becomes impossible in most cases. You will crave sugar and when your blood sugar is out of balance, you can get yeast overgrowths; eventually, you become resistant to insulin and excess glucose turns into fats.

That leaves you feeling worse than before and you may want to eat more sugary foods to boost your mood which may cause food cravings, mood swings, weight gain and fatigue.

Processed Foods

The processing of foods changes the original food and proportions of the nutrients within these foods. Pre-packaged and plastic-wrapped foods, quick fix, microwave, fast and boil in the bag type foods have gone through a multitude of processes before they end up in the supermarket. These foods have no nutritional value and years of eating bad carbohydrates could lead to diabetes. These processed foods can cause allergic reactions and stress on the liver to process such chemicals, many of which can cause cancer. Children exposed to processed foods can become hyperactive and display learning difficulties.

Prevention

The World Health Organization in 2016, confirmed that lifestyle changes could prevent type 2 diabetes; when patients lose weight by 7% to 10% it cuts the risk of diabetes by half. Consuming monounsaturated fats such as eating the Nordic diet, a low-carbohydrate diet was compared to slimming diets in most studies carried out in clinical trials. Drinking alcohol in moderation, taking a walk for twenty minutes every day and stopping smoking could reduce the risk of type 2 diabetes by a third.

Further, the latest findings in Diabetes Remission Clinic trials (DiRECT) published by the American Diabetes Association in 2019, also noted that losing five to ten per cent of your body weight can reverse type 2 diabetes. The study carried out at the University of Newcastle in 2019 by Dr Roy Taylor, a professor of Medicine in the UK, reassured patients that type 2 diabetes does not have to be a life sentence, people have choices of making small changes that are going to make big differences. By preventing food-related health problems such as diabetes by eating a low-calorie diet such as one packet of semi-skimmed milk or water per meal with non-starchy vegetables, will make people lose 3 kg on average in a week and they will be healthier and happy. The individual has got to want it and it is not the doctor's responsibility; it has to be cultural possible to individuals. The relationship between food and health is vital for us all.

The British Diabetes association added that eating a low carbohydrate diet prevents metabolic diseases such as high blood pressure, type 2 diabetes, dementia, renal failure, some types of cancer, stroke, and heart diseases. An investigation published by Lancet reported that people who reduced their calorie intake by 300 calories a day showed improvements in blood sugar levels, reduced body fat and weight loss.

Chapter 5: Benefits of and side effects of Ketones

The ketogenic diet or keto is a low-carbohydrate diet of about 20-50grams per day, with high fat, moderate protein and plenty of vegetables. It has been popular in the last decade due to the successful short-term health benefits of weight loss and improving other health conditions. Reducing carbohydrates to 20 grams per day causes the body to burn fat for fuel. This can put the body in a metabolic state known as (ketosis). Health professionals give warnings regarding the long-term effects of eating low carbohydrates and a large amount of fat.

In the United States and the rest of the world, patients noticed that this diet improves type 2 diabetes or metabolic syndrome. However, researchers suggest that a low-carbohydrate diet was not sustainable and should be considered for a short term. Eating low carbohydrates for three months, followed by a moderate carbohydrate of 130-230 grams per day was advised.

The benefits of a healthy ketogenic diet include weight loss, improved cardiovascular health, insulin sensitivity, reversing type 2 diabetes, improved cognitive performance, neuroprotection, reduces fatigue and blood sugar glucose is reduced. Consuming ketogenic foods provides all nutrients your body requires for health. People with type 2 diabetes should stay away from any type of sugar or anything that turns quickly into sugar such as corn, rice, wheat, and most fruits.

When you consume sugar, your body will burn it as fuel, and you will not experience the healthy weight loss benefits of fat burning. Carbohydrates raise blood sugar much more than protein and fat. However, there is little research on the benefits of the keto diet for other conditions such as acne, cancer, epilepsy, and polycystic ovary syndrome (PCOS).

Improve fatty liver disease

In non-alcoholic fatty liver disease (NAFD) a lot of fat is stored in the liver and the pancreas. I personally was able to reverse moderate fat liver through the process of eating a low-carbohydrate diet and by taking choline supplements at 250 mg twice a day for a period of two months. It is an essential nutrient for liver health. In addition, recent research supports that the keto diet may help reduce or reverse non-alcoholic fatty liver disease.

Possible side effects of the ketogenic diet

The keto diet has side effects such as headaches, fatigue, bad breath, stomach upset, sugar cravings, muscle cramps, raised cholesterol, brain fog and kidney stones. These side effects are rare; they may vary with the foods eaten, and low carbohydrates eaten for the long term may cause vitamin and mineral deficiencies.

Supplements

It has been observed that Chromium supplements, also known as glucose tolerance factor (GTF), will prevent and treat diabetes as well as hypoglycemia. All supplements are available at any health food store such as Holland & Barrett, Amazon, and many other online stores, like credenceonline.co.uk, OceanAlive.co.uk and others around the world. I have no connection to or am an affiliate of these companies. Supplements don't need to be prescribed because they are safe to take. Vanadium supplement replaces insulin in type 2 diabetes. Therefore, include chromium/vanadium at 250 mcg per day in your regime for prevention.

People with type 2 diabetes need an additional amino acid (protein) called L-arginine 1,000 mg - 3,000mg to be taken twice a day on an empty stomach. It has been shown to improve blood sugar, support heart health, reduce blood pressure, help the kidneys remove waste products from the body, maintain immune and hormone function, dilate and relax arteries and improve blood flow in arteries of the heart; it may help with erectile dysfunction because it improves blood flow and supports athletic performance. You can also obtain it through diet by consuming animal protein and some plant-based proteins such as almonds, lentils, black beans, peas, chickpeas, broccoli, cauliflower, and cabbage to name a few.

Studies have shown that L-arginine increases nitric oxide; it causes an increase in insulin sensitivity allowing better blood sugar control.

However, you should not take L-arginine supplements if you have cold sores or genital herpes; too much L-arginine in your system can activate the virus, and it can worsen asthma.

To help manage type 2 diabetes, include zinc 40-50 mg per day, take vitamin B12 1,000 mcg per day, quercetin supplements taken at 150 mg every day and glutathione supplements at 100mg per day. For as long as it takes until you feel well. Supplements are beneficial to our health with no side effects (most of them). Add supplements with betaine HCl and digestive enzymes of 75-200 mg per day before meals. It is always advisable to request a doctor for a blood test to check your blood sugar levels after three months of taking the above supplements. Individuals may not have to take all the suggested supplements, it all depends on an individual's condition. If your blood sugar levels are back to normal range, then your doctor may suggest that you don't have to take prescribed medication when it may not be necessary, and which may have side effects in most cases.

Resveratrol is a compound that is got from red grapes mainly. It is not just an anti-ageing supplement; resveratrol supplement has many health benefits such as lowering blood sugar levels in pre-diabetes and diabetes patients. Some exciting animal research has shown that resveratrol supplements can lower cholesterol, protect against clots, and protect the heart and circulatory system. There is evidence resveratrol may slow the progression of diabetes in kidney disease, which is a complication that can occur with both type 1 and type 2 diabetes.

Resveratrol reduces inflammation which puts people at higher risk of diabetes; studies have shown that resveratrol supplements can improve insulin sensitivity. Resveratrol supplements should be kept in a cool dark place, and it is best to take 2 capsules after eating a meal with fats. Have patience, it may take 60-90 days to heal.

Herbs & Spices

Astragalus root is traditional Mongolian medicine. It treats diabetes, lowers blood pressure, and protects the liver; it will give you energy and boost the immune system. Cinnamon tea will balance your blood sugar. Cinnamon essential oil relieves diabetes by reducing blood glucose levels; it supports the pancreas, helps in weight loss and in prevention and management of diabetes. Taking cinnamon supplements appears to be more effective in all forms of lowering blood sugar. Fenugreeks, cumin, and oregano essential oils blend are able to improve insulin sensitivity when taken internally. They can be taken in capsules or recipes.

Melissa essential oil regulates glucose when applied on the skin as aroma therapy. Berberine supplements 1,000mg per day reduce blood sugar and cholesterol levels. The best way to tackle diabetes is never to develop it in the first place; so, the best cure is prevention. You may have heard the saying by Benjamin Franklin that an ounce of prevention is worth a pound of cure. Other foods that enhance good health include Jerusalem artichoke and liquorice spirulina in liquid supplement or capsule form. The latter contains minerals like magnesium, potassium, manganese, chromium and adds colloidal minerals as it improves general well-being.

Chapter 6: Wrap up

Whatever you decide to do, try to use the information you've learned here. You don't have to use everything in this book; my hope is that you use it as a guidebook that you can come back to for some answers for the rest of your life and your family. People with type 2 diabetes should follow nutritional health advice by changing their lifestyles and consuming a low-carbohydrate diet for as long as it takes. Research confirms that type 2 diabetes is increased by eating refined carbohydrates in most cases.

In 2019, the United Nations insisted that maintenance of healthier dietary behaviour was necessary in order to improve the quality of life of people with type 2 diabetes and to decrease mortality from metabolic diseases such as cancer, high blood pressure and heart diseases. Prevention, treatment and weight management are essential.

There are many people in the world undiagnosed with type 2 diabetes which puts them at risk of developing other chronic diseases and causes financial losses. Too much alcohol puts strain on the digestive system and the liver and can lead to blood sugar imbalances and obesity.

The World Health Organization urges people to eat 25-29 grams of fibre daily. It reduces the risk of developing type 2 diabetes, stroke, colorectal cancer and coronary heart disease. Please pick a few things and decide what you are going to take action on, or whom you are going to help.

Some smart people spend their entire lives saving for their retirement years only to find that when the time comes, health is the new wealth. Hopefully, your personal portfolio is robust with this investment and your interest is compounding. However, even if it isn't, there is still time to change your lifestyle. Remember age doesn't cause you to become sick or feeble; decline is a function of how you choose to live. Therefore, keep educating yourselves and continue to develop. Your knowledge could change a life, in some cases save it. Do not lose hope. Type 2 diabetes can be reversed by constant lifestyle changes.

Bibliography

American Diabetes Association, "Standards of Medical Care in Diabetes. 2018 *Diabetes care; 41 (suppl):* S1. Available at: https://www.mayoclinic.org/diseases-conditions/diabetes/diagnosis-treatment/drc-20371451 accessed on: 20/Aug/ 2022

Ball. L., Davmor, R., Leveritt, M., Desbrow, B., Ehrlich, C., Chaboyer, "The nutrition care needs of patients newly diagnosed with type 2 diabetes: information dietetic practice". J.*Hum.Nutri. Diet* 2006, 29:487-494. Available at: https://pubmed.ncbi.nlm.nih.gov/26785827/ accessed on: 22nd / August/2022.

Casagrande, S.S., Cowie, C.C., "Trends in dietary intake among adults with type 2 diabetes NHNES 1988-2012". J. Hunter Diet, 2017;30:479. Available at: https://onlinelibrary.wiley.com/doi/10.1111/jhn.12443 accessed on:25th /August /2022

Dyson, P.A., Kelly, T., Duncan, A. Frost., G. Harrison, Z., Diabetes UK, evidence-based nutritional guidelines for prevention and management of diabetes, *Diabet Med.* 2011:28:1282-1288. Available at: https://pubmed.ncbi.nlm.nih.gov/21699560/ accessed on: 26th /August/2022.

Evert, A.B., Dennison, M., Gardener, C.C, Garvey, W.T., Lau, K.H.K., Macleod, J., Mitri, J Pereira., R.F.,

Rawlings, K., Robinson, S., et al. Nutrition Therapy for Adults with Diabetes or Prediabetes: A Consensus Report. Diabetes Care. 2019; 42:731-754.doi:10.2337/dci9 0014. Available at: https://www.ncbi.nlm.nih.gov/pmc/articles/PMC7011201/accessed on 3rd September /2022.

Gross, L.S., Li.L., Ford, E.S., Liu. S, "Increased consumption of refined Carbohydrates and Epidemic of type 2 Diabetes in the United States"; Ecologic Assessment. A.M.J, Clin.Nutr,2004;79;774-9, Available at: https://www.pubmed.ncbi.nlm.nih.gov/15113714/ accessed on 5th September 2022.

Index